Published By Adam Gilbin

@ Charles Garner

I0096750

Belly Diet: A Step by Step Diet Plan for Losing

Belly Fat to Achieve Your Go

ISBN 978-1-990666-86-5

TABLE OF CONTENTS

Easy Avocado Egg Salad

Ingredients:

- 3 slices bacon, crumbled

- 1 egg, hardboiled (diced)

- Sea salt

- Black pepper

- 1/2 avocado

- Juice from 1/2 a lemon

Directions:

1. Mash the avocado.
2. Drizzle with lemon juice.
3. Add the bacon to the avocado, mix gently to combine.
4. Add diced, hardboiled egg.

5. Season with sea salt and black pepper.

6. Enjoy!

Banana Almond Pancakes

Ingredients:

- 1/4 cup nuts of choice, (almonds, macadamia, or walnuts), chopped

- 2 tablespoon almond butter

- 1/4 teaspoon sea salt

- 1 1/2 teaspoon coconut oil

- 2 bananas, medium

- 1 1/2 tablespoon coconut flour

- 3 eggs

- 1 cup blueberries, fresh or frozen

Directions:

1. Mash bananas in a bowl.
2. Add the coconut flour, eggs, blueberries, nuts, and almond butter and salt, and blend well.
3. Heat a large nonstick skillet over medium heat, then apply a small pat of coconut oil to it.
4. Add small discs of batter to the hot pan.
5. Flip when batter loses its "tackiness" around the edges.
6. Cook other side over medium heat until well cooked.
7. Reapply coconut oil to the pan after each round of pancakes.

BBQ DoubleVeggie Burger Bowl

Ingredients:

- 1 bundle Boca Meatless Ground Burger

- 1 tablespoon grill sauce

- ½ cup frozen blended vegetables

Directions:

1. Place frozen veggies in a bowl; microwave for 1 moment on high.
2. Add Boca Meatless Ground Burger and microwave for an additional 2 minutes or until everything is hot.
3. Stir in grill sauce and enjoy!

Toasted Cheese and Turkey Sandwich

Ingredients:

- 3 cuts sans fat American cheddar

- 2 cuts simmered shop turkey

- 2 cuts lightwheat bread

Directions:

1. Toast bread in toaster oven or toaster oven oven.
2. Place cheddar and turkey between bread.
3. Microwave for 20 to 30 seconds.
4. Enjoy with an entire piece of fruit.

Mediterranean Egg Scramble Wraps

Ingredients:

- ¼ teaspoon kosher salt

- 2 tablespoons minced green onions

- 2 tablespoons diced roasted red peppers

- ¾ cup crumbled feta cheese

- ½ teaspoon oregano

- ¼ cup light sour cream

- 6 eggs

- ¼ teaspoon garlic powder

- 3 ground black peppercorns

- ½ teaspoon basil

- Flour tortillas or Crepes

Directions:

1. Preheat the skillet over medium heat.
2. Whisk the eggs, salt, sour cream, oregano, pepper, garlic powder, and basil together.
3. Now add in the crumbled feta cheese slowly into the mixture.
4. Once the skillet is hot, add butter then add the eggs and allow them to set up then scrape the bottom of your pan in order to let the liquid parts to cook.
5. Stir in the green onions and red peppers then cook until desired d2ness.
6. Serve immediately in crepes or flour tortillas, sprinkle some little feta cheese, then wrap.

Salmon Stuffed with Spinach

Ingredients:

- 2 cups fatfree lowsodium vegetable stock

- 1 teaspoon dried mint

- Salt and pepper to taste

- Juice of 1 lemon

- 2 tablespoons extra virgin olive oil, divided

- 4 salmon fillets with skin (3.5 ounces each)

- 2 tablespoons crumbled reducedfat feta cheese

- 1 (16ounce) bag frozen spinach, thawed and drained

Directions:

1. Preheat oven to 350 degrees F then heat a tablespoon of olive oil in a pan over medium heat.

2. Add the spinach then stir in order to coat with the olive oil then add feta cheese, pepper, mint and salt then stir to combine and remove from the heat.

3. Grease the bottom of a baking dish with the rest of the olive oil then place fillets on a work surface and cover with ½ cup of the spinach mixture on every fillet.

4. Roll the fillets up, place them in the baking dish and turn to coat with the olive oil.

5. Season with pepper and salt then pour the vegetable stock into the baking dish and pour the lemon juice over the fillets.

6. Cover with foil and bake until the salmon is cooked through.

7. This should take around 20 minutes.

Stuffed Peppers

Ingredients:

- ½ cup onion, slashed

- 1 cup cilantro, slashed

- 1 tsp. stew powder

- 2 tsp. cumin

- 8 sweet chime peppers

- 500 g. turkey, ground

- 100 g. green chillies, diced

- Salt

Directions:

1. Blend all the fixings in a medium dish, with the exception of the sweet chime peppers.
2. Cut off the highest point of the ringer peppers and put aside.
3. Stuff the bigger 50% of the peppers with the turkey mixture.
4. Place the stuffed ringer peppers in a preparing dish and spread with the tops that was situated aside.
5. Heat for 60 minutes at a 350 degree temperature. Serve while hot.

Turkey Club Sandwich

Ingredients:

- 1 cluster romaine lettuce

- 1 avocado, cut

- Dijon mustard 500 g.

- 2 cuts basic bread as explained earlier

- turkey breast, broiled

Directions:

1. Toast the basic bread cuts. On 2 bread cut, spread on the Dijon mustard.
2. Place 3 or more cuts of avocados.
3. Put on the lettuce, then 3 or three cuts of the simmered turkey.
4. Spread with the other bread cut.
5. Serve with your favourite sauce.

Delicious Dinner Chicken

Ingredients:

- 4 teaspoons of olive oil

- fresh juice from 2 lemons

- 2 tablespoons of fresh parsley, chopped

- 2 teaspoons of minced capers

- 2 kg chicken breast, skinless and b2less

- 2 tablespoons of flour

- Black pepper

Directions:

1. Place the chicken breasts on a flat working surface and work on them until they are totally flat.

2. Pass them onto the flour.

3. Over mediumhigh heat, place a large pan and add in the oil.

4. Heat it until it is sizzling. Now place your chicken in the pan and cook for about 3 minutes on each side or until it is lightly brown and well cooked.

5. Put in lemon juice, capers and the parsley and slowly boil.

6. Turn the heat down and simmer for 2 minutes in order to let the flavors to mix well.

7. Season your chicken with pepper for a good taste, then serve it with its juices.

Pita Sandwich with Olives and Turkey

Ingredients:

- 1 teaspoon of balsamic vinegar

- Sprinkling of red chilli

- 1 whole wheat pita cut in 1

- 100 grams of delisliced turkey breast.

- 8 green olives, pitted and chopped

- 8 green olives, pitted and chopped

- 1 teaspoon of olive oil

- I pack of mixed greens

Directions:

1. In a small bowl, combine the black and the green olives, vinegar, the red pepper flakes and oil.
2. Fill up each 1 of the pita with 1 of the turkey breast, greens and the olives.

Pancakes with Banana and Nutty H2y

Ingredients:

- A cup of skimmed milk

- Water An egg

- A tablespoon of canola oil

- A teaspoon of vanilla extract

- 2 large banana, cut into small pieces

- 2 tablespoons of fresh raspberries

- 1 cup basic pancake mix

- Pinch of ground cinnamon

- For walnut h2y, you will need 1/2 cup of chopped walnuts, 1/3 cup of h2y and a tablespoon of water.

Directions:

1. In a large bowl, make the pancake mix with cinnamon.
2. Mix together the buttermilk, oil, egg, water and the vanilla in another bowl.
3. Whisk them with the pancake mix and combine until you get a smooth mixture.
4. Fold the banana in, then set aside.
5. Using another small bowl, and mix together the h2y, walnuts and water.
6. Put a thin lining on a large pan with some cooking spray and add 2 spoon of pancake mix at a time to cook.
7. Make a few pancakes with the batter and once they are fully cooked, serve with the nutty h2y and some raspberry on the side.

Butternut Squash Soup with Curry

Ingredients:

- 4 cups fresh chopped butternut squash

- 4 cups chicken or vegetable broth

- 1 teaspoon fresh chopped thyme

- Fresh ground pepper

- 1 tablespoon olive oil

- 2 medium carrots, peeled and chopped

- 1 stalk celery, sliced

Directions:

1. Heat the oil in a large saucepan over mediumhigh heat.

2. Add the carrots and celery then cook for 4 minutes.
3. Stir in the butternut squash, broth, thyme and pepper then bring the mixture to a boil.
4. Reduce heat and simmer for 25 to 30 minutes until the squash is tender.
5. Remove from heat and puree the soup using an immersion blender. Serve hot.

Simple Chicken Piccata

Ingredients:

- ¼ cup olive oil

- 3 tablespoons fresh chopped parsley

- 2 tablespoons fresh lemon juice

- 1 tablespoon chopped capers

- 1 lbs. b2less skinless chicken tenders

- 2 tablespoons wholewheat flour

- Fresh ground pepper

Directions:

1. Sandwich the chicken tenders between pieces of parchment and pound them to ¼inch thick.
2. Toss the chicken tenders with the flour.

3. Heat the oil in a large skillet over mediumhigh heat.
4. Add the chicken and cook for 2 minutes on each side until evenly browned.
5. Add the parsley, lemon juice and capers and bring to a boil.
6. Reduce heat and simmer for a few minutes.
7. Season the chicken to taste with fresh ground pepper.

Cinnamon rubbed salmon with couscous & harissa yogurt

Ingredients:

- 1 tsp ground cinnamon , plus a large pinch

- 200ml hot vegetable stock

- 1 tbsp h2y

- 1 tbsp olive oil

- 2 salmon fillets

- 1 heaped tbsp harissa paste

- 100g couscous

- 2 tbsp sultanas

- small bunch coriander , chopped

- 170g tub 0% fat Greek yogurt

Directions:

1. Heat the grill. Put the couscous, sultanas, most of the coriander, 1 tsp cinnamon and some seasoning in a bowl.
2. Pour over the hot vegetable stock and set aside for 5 mins to soak.
3. Mix together the pinch of cinnamon, honey and oil.
4. Sit the salmon in a baking tray, spread over the honey mixture and season.
5. Cook under a hot grill for about 8 mins until the fish is cooked through.
6. Meanwhile, swirl together the harissa and yogurt.
7. Fluff up the couscous with a fork and serve with the fish and yogurt, sprinkled with the remaining coriander alongside some green beans, if you like.

Chicken & leek pot pies

Ingredients:

- 1 tbsp olive oil

- 4 leeks , sliced

- grated zest 1 lemon

- 2 tbsp chopped parsley

- 2 tbsp lowfat crème fraîche

- 1 tbsp wholegrain mustard

- 500g parsnip , peeled

- 300g floury potato , peeled

- 500g b2less skinless chicken breast

- 2 tsp cornflour

Directions:

1. Heat oven to 200C/fan 180C/gas 6.

2. Chop the parsnips and potatoes into chunks, then boil for 15 mins until tender.

3. Drain, reserving the water, then mash with a little seasoning.

4. Cut chicken into small chunks, then toss in the cornflour.

5. Heat the oil in a large pan, add the leeks, then fry for 3 mins until starting to soften.

6. Add the chicken and 200ml water from the potatoes, then bring to the boil, stirring.

7. Reduce the heat, then gently simmer for 10 mins, until the chicken is just tender.

8. Remove from the heat, then stir in the lemon zest, parsley, crème fraîche and mustard.

9. Divide the chicken filling between four 300ml pie dishes.

10. Spoon over the mash and spread roughly with a fork to seal in the filling. Bake for 25 mins until the topping is crisp and golden.

Lemon Cupcakes with Citrus Icing

Ingredients:

Cupcakes:

- 1/4 tsp salt

- 3/4 cup safflower oil

- 2 eggs

- 1/3 cup fatfree milk

- 1/4 cup freshly squeezed lemon juice

- 1 tsp freshly grated lemon zest

- 1 tsp lemon extract

- 1/2 tsp vanilla extract

- 1 2/3 cups unbleached allpurpose flour

- 1 cup sugar

- 2 tsp baking powder

- 1/2 tsp baking soda

Icing

- 2 Tbsp freshly squeezed orange juice

- 1 tsp freshly grated orange zest

- 1½ cups confecti2rs' sugar

Directions:

1. Preheat oven to 350°F. Line a 12cup muffin pan with paper liners.
2. Prepare the cupcakes: Combine the flour, sugar, baking powder, baking soda, and salt in a bowl.

3. Combine the oil, eggs, milk, lemon juice, lemon zest, lemon extract, and vanilla extract in a separate bowl.

4. Add to the flour mixture and stir until smooth.

5. Spoon the batter into the muffin cups and bake for 17 to 19 minutes or until lightly golden and the cupcakes are springy when gently touched.

6. Place pan on a rack and let cool for 5 minutes.

7. Remove the cupcakes from the pan, transfer to the rack, and let cool completely.

8. Prepare the icing: Combine the confectioners' sugar, orange juice, and orange zest in a bowl and stir until smooth.

9. Spread some of the glaze over each cupcake with a small spatula and let stand for at least 10 minutes before serving.

MapleCumin Tofu with Farro

Ingredients:

- 1 tablespoon olive oil

- 1 8ounce block of super extra firm tofu, cubed

- 2 tablespoons tamari (or soy sauce)

- 1/4 teaspoon fresh minced ginger (or ground ginger)

- 1/2 teaspoon garlic powder

- 1/2 teaspoon cumin

- 1 mediumsized carrot

- 1 cup farro

- 3 cups lowsodium vegetable broth

- 1 can black beans, rinsed

- 1 tablespoon maple syrup

- 1 red bell pepper, sliced

- 1 small crown of broccoli, cut into florets (about 2 cups)

Directions:

1. Add the farro and veggie broth to a covered pot.
2. Cook on high until boiling, reduce to simmer, and cook for another 30 minutes or until the farro is tender.
3. Stir in the black beans.
4. While the farro is cooking, place a large sauté pan on medium heat.
5. Add the olive oil, and allow it to heat up for a minute or so.

6. Add the tofu and drizzle with the tamari, and sprinkle with ginger, garlic powder, and cumin.
7. Use a spatula to stir it all up.
8. Allow the tofu to cook, stirring every couple minutes.
9. While the tofu is cooking, peel the carrots with a grater.
10. Then continue grating each carrot, creating long strips (they're much more fun to eat than chopped carrots).
11. After the tofu has cooked for 15 minutes, stir in the maple syrup.

12. Then add the carrots and bell peppers, and cook for 5 minutes.
13. Stir in the broccoli, and cook for another 10 minutes or until the broccoli looks vibrantly green and is slightly tender.

14. Spoon out 1/4 of the farrobean mixture into a bowl.
15. Top with 1/4 of the tofuveggie mixture, and enjoy immediately.

AlmondCranberry Quinoa Cookies

Ingredients:

- 1/4 cup (packed) light brown sugar

- 1/4 cup honey

- 2 large eggs

- 1 tea spoon vanilla extract

- 1/2 tea spoon almond extract

- 1 cup cooked quinoa, cooled

- 1 cup oldfashi2d oats

- 1 cup dried cranberries

- 1 1/2 cups white whole wheat flour

- 1 tea spoon kosher salt

- 1/2 tea spoon baking powder

- 1/2 tea spoon baking soda

- 1/2 cup (1 stick) unsalted butter, room temperature

- 1/4 cup sugar

- 1/2 cup slivered unsalted almonds

Directions:

1. Preheat oven to 375°. Line 2 baking sheets with parchment paper.
2. Whisk flour, salt, baking powder, and baking soda in a medium bowl.
3. Using an electric mixer, beat butter, both sugars, and honey in a large bowl until light and fluffy, about 3 minutes.
4. Add eggs and extracts; beat until pale and fluffy, about 2 minutes.
5. Beat in flour mixture, 1/2 cup at a time.

6. Stir in quinoa, oats, cranberries, and almonds.

7. Spoon dough in 2tablespoon portions onto prepared sheets, spacing 1" apart.

8. Bake cookies until golden, 12–15 minutes.

9. Transfer cookies to a wire rack and let cool.

10. DO AHEAD: Store cooled cookies airtight at room temperature for 1 day, or freeze for up to 1 month.

Red Quinoa with Pistachios

Ingredients:

- 1 cup quinoa, preferably red, rinsed well in a finemesh sieve

- 1 1/2 cups lowsodium chicken broth or water

- 1/4 cup unsalted, shelled raw pistachios, chopped

- 3 table spoons chopped flatleaf parsley

- 1 table spoon chopped fresh mint

- 1 table spoon olive oil

- 1 shallot, finely chopped

- Kosher salt and freshly ground black pepper

Directions:

1. Heat oil in a medium saucepan over medium heat.
2. Add shallot, season with salt and pepper, and cook, stirring occasionally, until soft, about 5 minutes.
3. Add quinoa and cook, stirring frequently, until quinoa starts to toast and smell nutty, about 5 minutes.
4. Add chicken broth and bring to a boil.
5. Stir in quinoa, reduce heat to low, cover, and simmer gently until quinoa is tender, 2530 minutes (15 if using white quinoa).
6. Remove pan from heat, fluff quinoa with a fork. Cover; let stand for 5 minutes.
7. Fold pistachios, parsley, and mint into quinoa. Season with salt and pepper.

Sunshine Smoothie

Ingredients:

- 2 cup of vanilla yogurt

- 2third cup of orange juice

- 2 tbsp. of h2y

- 3 nectarines (pitted, quartered)

- 2 banana (cut in chunks)

- 2 orange (peeled, quartered)

Directions:

1. Add banana chunks, nectarines, and orange in a blender. Blender for 3 minutes.
2. Add vanilla yogurt, h2y, and orange juice. Blend the Ingredients: until frothy and smooth.

41

3. Pour the smoothie in glasses and serve.

Mango Kale Berry Smoothie

Ingredients:

- 1 cup of mango chunks

- 2fourth cup of water

- 3 tbsps. of chia seeds

- 2 cup of orange juice

- 2third cup of kale

- 2 and a 1 cup of mixed berries (frozen)

Directions:

1. Take a high power blender and add kale, orange juice, berries, mango chunks, chia seeds, and 1 a cup of water.

2. Blend the Ingredients: on high settings until smooth.
3. In case the smoothie is very thick, you can adjust the consistency by adding more water.
4. Pour the smoothie in glasses and serve.

Dreamy Macaroni & Cheese Style Spaghetti Squash

Ingredients:

- 1 tablespoon frozen peas

- 1 cut green pepper (finely diced)

- ¼ cup destroyed cheddar (TexMex blend)

- 1 tablespoon destroyed Parmesan cheese

- 1 finely diced green onion

- 1 ½ cups cooked spaghetti squash

- ½ tablespoon of wheat free flour (coconut, almond, rice, flax seed feast to name a few)

- ¼ cup 1% milk

- Salt and pepper

Directons:

1. Preheat stove to 350 degrees. Utilizing cooking shower, splash the base and the sides of a goulash dish and set aside.
2. In a pot (little), whisk flour, salt, and pepper together, over medium heat.
3. Add in milk gradually until the blend becomes smooth.
4. Mix and cook until combination thickens.
5. Remove from hotness and add the destroyed TexMex mix cheddar.
6. Mix until smooth and completely melted.
7. Pour cheddar sauce over the spaghetti squash and consolidate well in a bowl.
8. Spread the combination onto the goulash dish.
9. Sprinkle the top with the onion, peas, green pepper, and Parmesan cheese.

10. Bake at 350 degrees for 20 minutes or until the cheddar has dissolved and the spaghetti squash has been warmed as far as possible through.

Spicy Burgers

Ingredients:

- 2 teaspoons olive oil

- 1 tablespoon garam masala (yes it is a genuine spice)

- 1 teaspoon ground cinnamon

- 1.7 ounces of slashed almonds

- 1 huge carrot, stripped and grated

- 1 lemon, ground (zest)

- 1 enormous egg, beaten

- Olive oil for frying

- 16 ounces of additional lean ground meat, sheep, or bison

- 1.7 ounces of breadcrumbs (wheat or glutenfree)

- 1 huge onion, finely chopped

- Freshly ground dark pepper

Directons:

1. In a huge skillet, heat the olive oil and add the onion until it turns out to be delicate and golden.
2. Add the cinnamon and garam masala and cook for about a moment.
3. Eliminate the container from hotness and tip the substance into a major bowl. Set the dish aside.
4. Add the ground sheep or meat, almonds, carrot, breadcrumbs, and the lemon zing to the bowl that contains the onion combination.

5. Consolidate the fixings well. Season with dark pepper and add the beaten egg. Blend well again.

6. Divide the combination into 8 sections, and shape each part into a burger.

7. Heat a limited quantity of olive oil in the container utilized beforehand.

8. Put the burgers on the dish and make certain to burn them rapidly on each side.

9. Remove them from the container and put on a baking plate (nonstick).

10. Bake the burgers for around 15 minutes or somewhere in the vicinity, until they are cooked through.

11. You can serve the burgers with a without wheat roll, with mango chutney and lettuce.

Basic Buckwheat Pasta Dough Recipe

Ingredients:

- 1 cup buckwheat flour

- 1 egg, beaten

- 2 tablespoons water (or as needed to moisten)

- 1/2 teaspoon salt (essential)

- 1/2 teaspoon oil

Directons:

1. In a medium mixing bowl, and the salt and flour.
2. Mix thoroughly. Make a well in the center and pour in the beaten egg.

3. If you have an electric mixer, use a dough hook at mediumlow speed to slowly mix the eggs into the flour. No mixer? Just use a fork.

4. Then turn the dough out onto a floured counter top.

5. Knead the dough, adding flour as needed an a little water until it is smooth and firm.

6. The pasta dough is d2 and ready to be shaped when you can place it on a clean surface (no flour) without it sticking.

7. Grease a bowl with the oil. Add the pasta dough and turn to coat the surface of the dough.

8. Divide the dough to create tennis sized balls.

9. Wrap each ball of pasta dough in plastic wrap and allow to rest at room temperature for 45 minutes (or longer)

10. This is a basic pasta recipe that lends itself well to adding basil, spinach, garlic powder or other flavorings.

11. Just remember to pass larger herbs, spices, etc. through a food processor so everything is chopped very fine.

12. Then mix them into the flour before adding the egg.

Homemade Buckwheat Soba recipe

Ingredients:

- ½ cup water

- ½ tablespoon fresh lemon juice

- 2 cups of buckwheat flour

Directons:

1. The night before, place the flour in a medium size bowl.
2. Pour the water and lemon juice into the bowl and mix with a wooden spoon until you've combined it.
3. It will most likely be a crumbly mixture at this point.
4. Using your hands, start kneading the mixture until the water and four starts turning into a ball.

5. Knead for a few minutes until it forms into a firm ball.

6. Place over the ball of dough to keep it moist while it "soaks".

7. Leave the bowl out on the counter top overnight for 12 24 hours.

8. Divide the dough into four sections.

9. Using arrowroot powder, buckwheat flour, or even white flour (only if you don't have to be gluten free), flour the rolling surface well.

10. Using a sharp knife, cut the noodles into 1/8 inch "slices" all the way down the dough.

11. Repeat this process with the rest of the dough and let the noodles rest for about 1020 minutes before cooking.

Simple Vegan Oatmeal

Ingredients:

- 2 tsp coconut or brown sugar

- 2 medium bananas

- 1/4 cup of Raspberries

- ½ cup rolled oats (60 g)

- 1 ½ cups plant milk of your choice

Directons:

1. Place the oats and the milk in a saucepan and cook over medium heat until the oats are cooked (10 to 15 minutes). Stir occasionally.
2. Serve the oatmeal in 3 bowls and add 2 Teaspoon of sugar in each bowl.
3. As the oatmeal is hot, the sugar will melt and it will look like a syrup.

4. Add 2 sliced banana in each bowl and raspberries to taste.

Blueberry Oatmeal Waffles

Ingredients:

- 1/4 teaspoon ground allspice

- 1 cup quick cooking oats

- 1/3 cup unsweetened applesauce

- 1 1/2 cups unsweetened almond milk (or your favourite nondairy milk)

- 3 tablespoons pure maple syrup

- 2 tablespoons canola oil

- 1 cup white whole wheat flour

- 1 tablespoon baking powder

- 1/2 teaspoon salt

- 1 teaspoon pure vanilla extract

Directons:

1. Sift flour, baking powder, salt and allspice into a mixing bowl.
2. Mix in the oats. Make a well in the center and add applesauce, milk, maple syrup, oil and vanilla.
3. Stir with just until combined.
4. Let batter rest for 5 minutes or so, it will thicken a bit.
5. Fold in the blueberries. Don't worry too much about the blueberries bleeding into the batter, it's no biggie.
6. Cook in waffle iron according to manufacturer Directions:.
7. Remember to spray or brush the iron with oil in between each waffle.

Simple Breakfast Muffins

Ingredients:

- 1/2 cup coconut flour

- 6 eggs

- 6 tablespoons coconut oil, melted

- 1 teaspoon vanilla extract

- 1 teaspoon baking powder

- Powdered stevia

- 1/4 teaspoon sea salt

- 1/2 cup frozen fruit

Directions:

1. Preheat oven to 400 degrees F.

2. Blend together all Ingredients: except frozen fruit.

3. Once Ingredients: are thoroughly mixed, fold in the frozen fruit.

4. Next, pour batter into muffin cups

5. Bake for 15 minutes.

Blueberry Coconut Sc2s

Ingredients:

- 6 oz fresh blueberries, organic

- 2 tablespoons cornstarch, or arrowroot powder

- 1/4 cup unrefined sugar

- 1 teaspoon vanilla

- 1 teaspoon baking powder, aluminum free

- 1 1/2 cups almond flour

- 1/4 cup shredded coconut, unsweetened

- 2 eggs, organic

- 1/4 cup coconut oil

Directons:

1. Line a 9" round baking pan with unbleached parchment paper. Set aside.
2. Combine the egg, coconut oil and sugar in a mixing bowl. Beat with a hand mixer until well mixed.
3. Add the remainder of the Ingredients: except the blueberries and mix thoroughly.
4. Add the blueberries and use your hands to incorporate them into the batter.
5. Press the batter into the prepared baking pan.
6. Bake in a preheated oven at 350 F for 3540 minutes.
7. Let the sc2s cool for at least 15 minutes.
8. Lift the sc2s up from the pan and cut into 8 pieces.

Mango Marinated Steak

Ingredients:

- 1/2 cup extra virgin olive oil

- 1/2 teaspoon red pepper flakes

- 1/4 teaspoon cayenne pepper

- 1/4 teaspoon black pepper

- 1 mango, diced

- 1 lb beef sirloin, cut into cubes

- Handful of cherry tomatoes

- 2 cloves garlic, minced

- 1 1/2 tablespoons balsamic vinegar

- 1 red onion, cut into chunks

- 1 red bell pepper, cut into chunks

Directions:

1. In a saucepan, combine garlic, vinegar, olive oil, red pepper flakes, cayenne pepper, and black pepper.
2. Cook over low heat for 5 minutes. Stir occasionally.
3. Add mango and continue to cook on low heat for an additional 4 6 minutes, stirring occasionally.
4. Remove from heat when mixture thickens.
5. Place steak in a glass dish and pour mango marinade over it.
6. Cover the dish and store in the refrigerator for a minimum of 2 hour.
7. Thread skewers with the marinated steak, tomatoes, onion, and bell peppers.
8. Place skewers on a hot grill and cook until d2.

Teriyaki Chicken Power Pita

Ingredients:

- 4 tablespoons diced tomatoes

- 2 teaspoons white onions, diced

- 2 tablespoons sweet peppers Dash of salt and pepper

- 1 enormous entire wheat pita

- 1 Simply Grilled Chicken Breast, cooked

- ½ cup slashed spring blend lettuce

- 2 tablespoons lowsodium teriyaki sauce

Directions:

1. Slice pita in 1.
2. Chop chicken bosom and blend in with different fixings in a bowl.

3. Evenly partition chicken combination and spot into discrete pita pockets.

Ultimate Veggie Wrap

Ingredients:

- 1 tablespoon green pepper slices

- ¼ cup horse feed sprouts

- 1 tablespoon destroyed carrots

- 1 tablespoon without fat disintegrated feta cheddar 1 tablespoon balsamic vinegar

- 1 12inch spinach tortilla

- ½ cup spinach leaves

- 1 tablespoon tomatoes, diced

- 1 tablespoon mushrooms, cut 1 tablespoon broiled red peppers

Directions:

1. Lay tortilla level on a plate.
2. Heap different fixings on top of tortilla. Fold tortilla into a wrap.

Roasted Vegetables with Lamb Cutlets

Ingredients:

- 8 lean lamb cutlets

- 1 red onion, cut into wedges

- 2 zucchinis, sliced into chunks

- 1 sweet potato, peeled and cut into chunks

- 1 tablespoon olive oil

- 2 green peppers deseeded and cut into chunky pieces

- 2 tablespoons chopped mint leaves

- 1 tablespoon chopped thyme leaf

Directions:

1. Preheat the oven to 425 degrees Fahrenheit then put the sweet potato, zucchini, onion and peppers in a large baking pan and drizzle with the olive oil then season with black pepper and roast these for 25 minutes.
2. In the meantime, trim the lamb of any fat then mix the herbs with black pepper and pat over the lamb.
3. Remove the vegetables from the oven, then turn over and then push to 2 side of the tray then put the cutlets on the other side then return to the oven and cook for ten minutes.
4. After the ten minutes, turn the cutlets then cook for another ten minutes or until the lamb and vegetables are tender.
5. Mix everything in the tray then serve.

Stuffed Portobello Mushrooms

Ingredients:

- 2 cups spinach, chopped

- Salt and pepper

- 1 tablespoon olive oil

- ½ onion, chopped

- ¼ cup goat cheese, crumbled

- 4 cloves garlic, minced

- 4 Portobello mushrooms

- ½ cup mozzarella cheese

- ½ green bell pepper, chopped

- 1 tablespoon hot sauce

- ½ cup bread crumbs

- 4 tomatoes, chopped

Directions:

1. Preheat the oven to 400 degrees Fahrenheit.
2. Remove the stems from the mushrooms carefully and put the mushrooms with the stem part facing down on the baking pan.
3. Bake for 1015 minutes until all the water leaks out then remove from the oven and use paper towels to soak the excess water then put aside.
4. Chop the mushroom stems to add to the stuffing.
5. Heat the olive oil in a skillet over medium heat and add the garlic and onion then sauté for several minutes until the onion is translucent.
6. Add the spinach and green pepper to the skillet and cook for several minutes then add

the goat cheese, tomatoes, mushroom stems, pepper, salt, breadcrumbs and hot sauce.

7. Stir to combine then cook for another few minutes.

8. Stuff the mushrooms with the mixture and top with mozzarella cheese then bake until the cheese melts.

9. This should take around ten minutes.

Pumpkin Pie Flan

Ingredients:

- ½ teaspoon ground nutmeg

- ½ cup whole milk

- 1 teaspoon ground cinnamon

- 1 teaspoon vanilla extract

- ¼ cup evaporated milk

- 2 large egg yolks

- 2 eggs

- ¾ cup canned solidpack pumpkin

- Nonstick cooking spray

- 2/3 cup granulated sugar

Directions:

1. Preheat the oven to 350 degrees Fahrenheit then arrange 8 (4ounce) ramekins in a baking pan then coat the ramekins with cooking spray.

2. Heat 1/3 cup of sugar in a pan over medium heat then stir constantly until it melts and forms a caramel.

3. This should take around 7 minutes. Transfer 3 teaspoons of the caramel to every ramekin then swirl immediately you spoon in the caramel into the ramekins then put aside.

4. Mix the evaporated milk and whole milk in a pan over medium heat until warm then reduce the heat and simmer then keep warm. In the meantime, bring four cups of water to a boil then keep hot.

5. Whisk together the egg yolks, eggs, remaining sugar, cinnamon, nutmeg and vanilla in a bowl then fold in the pumpkin.

6. Fold the pumpkin mixture into the warm milk mixture and divide among the 8 ramekins and place in a baking pan in the oven.

7. Pour hot water into the baking pan until 1way then bake for around 35 minutes or until they just set then allow to cool completely.

8. Place a dessert plate on top of every ramekin then invert and the flan will slide out with the syrup overflowing on the sides.

Delicious Fish Sticks

Ingredients:

- 6 tbsp. Olive oil

- 1 cup almond flour

- 1/2 kg. White fish fillet

- 2 eggs

- Salt

Directions:

1. Flush the cuts of fish and place on a plate. Uproot the b2s of the fish and cut into 1 by 5 inch rectangles.
2. Blend the flour and salt in 2 bowl, the eggs in a different dish.

3. Dunk the fish into the eggs in the first place, then into the flour rapidly. Set up all the fish in this way on a plate.

4. Over medium warmth, warm a pan with three tablespoons of olive oil.

5. Place 50% of the fish fillets on the pan sufficiently leaving space to turn them over and cook.

6. Cook every side of the fish until chestnut. Serve with your favourite sauce or ketchup.

Glazed Pork Tenderloin

Ingredients:

- 2 tablespoons coconut oil, additional virgin olive oil, or butter

- ¼ cup beef puree

- 1 tablespoon balsamic vinegar

- 2 tablespoons Dijon mustard

- 1 pound pork tenderloin

- 1 teaspoon ground cardamom

- ½ teaspoon ground dark pepper

- ¼ teaspoon ocean salt

Directions:

1. Preheat the oven to 350°F.
2. On a work surface, rub the tenderloin uniformly with the cardamom, pepper, and salt.
3. In a heatproof heating pan or oven proof skillet over mediumhigh warmth, warm the oil.
4. Cook the tenderloin, turning at times, for 8 minutes, or until sautéed on all sides. Place in the oven.
5. Cook for 20 minutes, or until a thermometer embedded in the middle registers 160°F and the juices run clear.
6. Expel from the oven and exchange the pork to a cutting board. Let stand for 10 minutes.
7. Place the skillet over mediumhigh warmth. Include the beef puree and vinegar. Heat to the point of boiling, mixing to uproot any cooked bits.

8. Cook until the mixture is decreased by about 1.

9. Rush in the mustard. Cut the pork and shower with the sauce.

Beaded Pork Chops

Ingredients:

- 1 teaspoon sans gluten soy sauce

- ½ cup ground pecans

- 4 b2less pork loin slashes, ¾" thick

- 2 tablespoons olive or coconut oil

- 2 tablespoons ground brilliant flaxseeds

- ½ teaspoon ocean salt

- ½ teaspoon smoked paprika

- 1 vast egg

Directions:

1. On a plate, join the flaxseeds, salt, and paprika. In a wide shallow dish, whisk the egg and soy sauce.
2. Place the pecans on a plate.
3. Dunk every hack into the flax mixture, then in the egg mixture, and after that into the pecans to coat.
4. In a huge skillet over mediumhigh warmth, warm the oil.
5. Cook the pork hacks for 8 minutes, turning once, or until a thermometer embedded sideways in a cleave registers 160°F and the juices run clear.

Grilled Balsamic Salmon Fillets

Ingredients:

- 1 tablespoon Dijon mustard

- Fresh ground pepper

- 2 lbs. b2less salmon fillet

- ½ cup olive oil

- ¼ cup balsamic vinegar

Directions:

1. Whisk together the marinade Ingredients: in a bowl.
2. Cut the salmon into 2inch chunks and place it in a shallow dish.
3. Pour the marinade over the salmon and turn to coat – let rest for 30 minutes.

4. Preheat the grill to high heat and brush the grates with oil.

5. Place the fillets on the grill upside down and cook for 2 to 3 minutes.

6. Flip the fillets and grill for 2 to 3 minutes until grill marks appear.

7. Close the lid and cook until the flesh of the fish flakes easily with a fork – don't overcook.

Turkey Meatloaf

Ingredients:

- 2 large eggs, whisked well

- 1 teaspoon dried oregano

- Fresh ground pepper

- 2 lbs. lean ground turkey

- ½ cup wholewheat breadcrumbs

- 1 small red pepper, cored and diced

Directions:

1. Preheat the oven to 375°F.
2. Combine all of the Ingredients: in a mixing bowl and stir well.
3. Turn out the mixture onto a parchmentlined baking sheet and shape into a loaf.

4. Bake for 50 to 60 minutes until the meatloaf is cooked through.
5. Cool the meatloaf on a cutting board for 10 minutes before slicing to serve.

Chicken & leek pot pies

Ingredients:

- 2 tsp cornflour

- 1 tbsp olive oil

- 4 leeks , sliced

- grated zest 1 lemon

- 2 tbsp chopped parsley

- 2 tbsp lowfat crème fraîche

- 1 tbsp wholegrain mustard

- 500g parsnip , peeled

- 300g floury potato , peeled

- 500g boneless skinless chicken breast

Directions:

1. Heat oven to 200C/fan 180C/gas 6.
2. Chop the parsnips and potatoes into chunks, then boil for 15 mins until tender.
3. Drain, reserving the water, then mash with a little seasoning.
4. Cut chicken into small chunks, then toss in the cornflour.
5. Heat the oil in a large pan, add the leeks, then fry for 3 mins until starting to soften.
6. Add the chicken and 200ml water from the potatoes, then bring to the boil, stirring.
7. Reduce the heat, then gently simmer for 10 mins, until the chicken is just tender.
8. Remove from the heat, then stir in the lemon zest, parsley, crème fraîche and mustard.
9. Divide the chicken filling between four 300ml pie dishes.
10. Spoon over the mash and spread roughly with a fork to seal in the filling.

11. Bake for 25 mins until the topping is crisp and golden.

Turkey & parsnip curry

Ingredients:

- 500g parsnip , peeled and cut into chunks

- 5 tbsp Madras curry paste

- 400g can chopped tomatoes

- 500g/1lb 2oz b2less cooked turkey , cut into chunks

- 150g pot lowfat natural yogurt

- 2 tbsp vegetable oil

- 2 onions , halved through the root and thinly sliced

- cooked basmati rice , to serve

Directions:

1. Heat the oil in a saucepan, add the onions and fry gently for 10 minutes until they are softened and lightly coloured.
2. Add the parsnips and stir well.
3. To make the curry, stir in the curry paste, then add the tomatoes with a little salt, and stir well.
4. Add 1½ canfuls of water and bring to the boil.
5. Reduce the heat, cover and simmer for 1520 minutes, until the parsnips are just tender.
6. To finish, stir in the turkey chunks, cover the pan again and simmer for a further 5 minutes until the turkey is heated through.
7. Remove from the heat. (The curry can now be cooled and frozen for up to 2 months.)
8. Lightly swirl in the yogurt and serve with basmati rice.

Quinoa Mason Jar Salads

Ingredients:

For the quinoa:

- 1 cup uncooked quinoa

- 2 cups vegetable broth

- For the sautéed tofu:

- 1 teaspoon olive oil

- 1 container super extra firm cubed tofu (7 ounces)

- 1 teaspoon garlic powder

- 1/2 teaspoon sea salt

For the salad:

- 10 tablespoons dressing (You can use Annie's Gingerly Vinaigrette)

- 2 1/2 cups black beans

- 1 red pepper, diced

- 2 cups shredded carrots

- 1 yellow pepper

- 5 stalks celery, sliced

- 1 cucumber, diced

- 1 1/4 cups red grapes, halved

- 5 cups mixed greens

- 5 tablespoons salted sunflower seeds

Directions:

1. Place the quinoa and veggie broth in a covered pot.
2. Heat on high until it starts to boil, then reduce heat to low and simmer for 20 minutes.
3. While the quinoa is cooking, add the olive oil to a cast iron pan and turn heat on to medium.
4. Add the cubed tofu, sprinkle with garlic powder and salt.
5. Stir every few minutes and saute for about 10 minutes, or until the edges are slightly browned.
6. While the quinoa and tofu are cooking, prep the beans and veggies.
7. Allow the quinoa and tofu to cool before adding to the mason jars.
8. To speed up this process, place them in separate bowls in the fridge for 10 minutes.

9. Start adding the ingredients to your mason jars.

10. Start with the dressing, then add the beans, quinoa, red pepper, carrots, yellow pepper, celery, cucumbers, grapes, greens, tofu, and sunflower seeds.

11. Secure each lid and store in the fridge.

12. Shake up the salad once you're ready to eat, or you can pour it into a large bowl if you prefer.

MapleCumin Tofu with Farro

Ingredients:

- 2 tablespoons tamari (or soy sauce)

- 1/4 teaspoon fresh minced ginger (or ground ginger)

- 1/2 teaspoon garlic powder

- 1/2 teaspoon cumin

- 1 mediumsized carrot

- 1 tablespoon maple syrup

- 1 red bell pepper, sliced

- 1 small crown of broccoli, cut into florets (about 2 cups)

- 1 cup farro

- 3 cups lowsodium vegetable broth

- 1 can black beans, rinsed

- 1 tablespoon olive oil

- 1 8ounce block of super extra firm tofu, cubed

Directions:

1. Add the farro and veggie broth to a covered pot.
2. Cook on high until boiling, reduce to simmer, and cook for another 30 minutes or until the farro is tender. Stir in the black beans.
3. While the farro is cooking, place a large sauté pan on medium heat.
4. Add the olive oil, and allow it to heat up for a minute or so.
5. Add the tofu and drizzle with the tamari, and sprinkle with ginger, garlic powder, and cumin.

6. Use a spatula to stir it all up.

7. Allow the tofu to cook, stirring every couple minutes.

8. While the tofu is cooking, peel the carrots with a grater.

9. Then continue grating each carrot, creating long strips (they're much more fun to eat than chopped carrots).

10. After the tofu has cooked for 15 minutes, stir in the maple syrup.

11. Then add the carrots and bell peppers, and cook for 5 minutes.

12. Stir in the broccoli, and cook for another 10 minutes or until the broccoli looks vibrantly green and is slightly tender.

13. Spoon out 1/4 of the farrobean mixture into a bowl. Top with 1/4 of the tofuveggie mixture, and enjoy immediately.

CuminScented Quinoa and Black Rice

Ingredients:

- 3 large garlic cloves, minced

- 2 tea spoons cumin seeds

- 3 table spoons fresh lemon juice

- 1/4 cup chopped fresh cilantro

- 1/4 cup chopped flatleaf parsley

- 2 table spoons 1' pieces chives

- Freshly ground black pepper

- 1 avocado, peeled, pitted

- 1 lemon, cut into wedges

- 1/2 cup shortgrain black rice

- 1 cup red quinoa, rinsed well

- 1 bay leaf

- 1/4 tea spoon kosher salt plus more

- 4 table spoons extravirgin olive oil, divided

- 1 small onion, finely chopped

Directions:

1. Bring rice and 1 cup water to a boil in a small saucepan.
2. Cover, reduce heat to low, and cook until water is absorbed and rice is tender, 25–30 minutes.
3. Meanwhile, combine quinoa, bay leaf, 1/4 tsp. salt, and 2 cups water in a medium saucepan.
4. Bring to a boil. Cover, reduce heat to low, and simmer until quinoa is tender, about 15 minutes.
5. Drain; return quinoa to hot saucepan.

6. Cover and let sit for 15 minutes. Discard bay leaf, fluff quinoa with a fork, and transfer to a large bowl.
7. Heat 2 Tbsp. oil in a large skillet over medium heat.
8. Add onion and cook, stirring occasionally, until soft, about 8 minutes.
9. Add garlic and cumin and cook, stirring often, for 2 minutes. Add to quinoa.
10. Add rice; mix well. Stir in remaining 2 Tbsp. oil, fresh lemon juice, cilantro, parsley, and chives.
11. Season to taste with salt and pepper. Cut avocado into wedges. Serve salad with avocado and lemon wedges.

Stellar Quinoa Burger

Ingredients:

- 1 small shallot, finely chopped

- ¼ tea spoon crushed red pepper flakes

- 1 cup cooked quinoa (from about ½ uncooked)

- ¾ cup dried breadcrumbs

- 1½ tea spoons fresh lemon juice

- 4 English muffins, split, toasted

- 1 small sweet potato

- 6 table spoons olive oil, divided

- Kosher salt, freshly ground pepper

- 1 portobello mushroom

- ½ small zucchini

- Guacamole, tomato chutney, and sprouts (for serving; optional)

Directions:

1. Preheat oven to 350°. Prick sweet potato all over with a fork; rub with 1 Tbsp. oil, then season with salt and pepper. Roast directly on oven rack until tender, 30–45 minutes. Let cool. Remove and discard skin; mash flesh with a fork. Set aside.
2. Remove stem from mushroom; discard.
3. Pulse cap in a food processor until finely chopped.
4. Coarsely grate zucchini on the large holes of a box grater; gather up in a kitchen towel and squeeze out excess liquid.
5. Heat 1 Tbsp. oil in a medium skillet over low.

6. Cook shallot and red pepper flakes, stirring often, until shallot is soft, about 2 minutes.

7. Add mushroom and zucchini and cook, stirring occasionally, until vegetables begin to release their liquid but have not taken on any color, about 2 minutes.

8. Transfer to a large bowl; mix in quinoa and season with salt and pepper. Let cool.

9. Add breadcrumbs, lemon juice, and about ¼ cup reserved mashed sweet potato to quinoa mixture and mix well.

10. Taste and adjust seasoning with salt and pepper if needed. If mixture is too loose, add more sweet potato to bind.

11. Divide mixture into 4 portions and form into patties, pressing firmly together with your hands. Heat 2 Tbsp. oil in a medium skillet over medium and cook 2 patties until golden brown, about 2 minutes per side; season with salt and pepper.

12. Repeat with remaining 2 Tbsp. oil and 2 patties.

13. Build burgers with patties, toasted English muffins, guacamole, tomato chutney, and sprouts.

14. Do Ahead: Patties can be made 3 days ahead. Cover and chill.

Breakfast Pink Smoothie

Ingredients:

- 3 carrots

- 3 cups of coconut milk (light)

- 2 small beet (quartered)

- 2 and a 1 cup of strawberries (frozen)

- 2 cup of raspberries

- 2 orange (peeled)

Directions:

1. Add strawberries, raspberries, and orange in a blender. Blend until frothy and smooth.
2. Add beet, carrots, and coconut milk.
3. Blend again for 2 minute.
4. Divide the smoothie in glasses and serve.

Butternut Squash Smoothie

Ingredients:

- 3 ripe bananas

- 2 tsp. of cinnamon (ground)

- 3 tbsps. of hemp protein

- 1 cup of strawberries

- 2 tbsp. of chia seeds

- 1 tbsp. of bee pollen

- 3 cups of almond milk

- 2fourth cup of nut butter (of your choice)

- 2 cup of water

- 2 and a 1 cup of butternut squash (frozen)

Directions:

1. Add butternut squash, bananas, strawberries, and almond milk in a blender. Blend until frothy and smooth.
2. Add water, nut butter, cinnamon, hemp protein, chia seeds, and bee pollen. Blend the Ingredients: f0r 3 minutes.
3. Divide the smoothie in glasses and enjoy!

Wheatfree Garlic Bread

Ingredients:

Wet:

- 1/3 cup of entire psyllium husks

- 1/3 cup of ground chia seeds

- 2 ½ cups of warm water (around 105110°F)

- 1 teaspoon h2y

- 2 tablespoons maple syrup

- 2 ¼ teaspoons of dynamic dry yeast

- 2 tablespoons of additional virgin olive oil (in addition to extra for topping)

Dry:

- 1 cup sorghum flour

- ½ cup sweet rice flour

- 1 cup teff flour

- ½ cup almond meal

- 1 ½ teaspoons of ocean salt

Directions:

1. Freshly cleaved garlic Poppy seeds Sesame seeds When you purchase entire chia seeds, utilize an espresso processor to crush them. Store the ground chia seeds in a glass container and pop it in the cooler just until a week.

2. Preheat the stove to 400° Fahrenheit. Put the warm water in a bowl.

3. Consolidate a teaspoon of h2y and the yeast and whisk them together.

4. Leave the blend for around 510 minutes to allow the yeast to actuate.

5. The combination ought to turn out to be effervescent or frothy.

6. In the event that this doesn't occur, dispose of the combination and start over.

7. While the yeast is being actuated, you can begin blending the dry fixings in a major bowl.

8. When the yeast is enacted, include the maple syrup, olive oil, psyllium husks, and ground chia seeds into the blend.

9. Leave the blend for around 23 minutes (this is significant, so watch an opportunity) to let the psyllium and the chia seeds discharge a gelatinlike substance. Whisk these together.

10. Pour every 2 of the wet fixings into the bowl with the dry fixings.

11. Combine everything as 2 utilizing a wooden spoon until the combination turns out to be thick.

12. On a floured wooden board, manipulate the batter to blend in the flour. Add the newly slashed garlic as you work. Add a greater amount of the sorghum and teff flours, a little at a time. Keep adding until the mixture keeps yet is still a piece tacky to the touch.

13. Make a ball with the batter and set it back into the enormous bowl. Cover it with a clammy towel.

14. Place the bowl in a warm spot with the goal that the batter rises. Some put the bowl on a pot that has warm water.

15. Allow it to ascend until the batter is multiplied in size.

16. When the mixture has risen, put a pizza st2 inside the broiler.

17. Set a container of water on the base rack, just underneath the pizza st2.

18. You can utilize a 8x8inch glass container loaded up with water (about ¾ of the way).

19. Punch the mixture down and spread it out onto a wooden board that has been gently floured. Ply it for about a moment and afterward structure it into a ball. Put the mixture on a square piece of material paper. Utilizing a sharp blade, make a shallow example on top (a spasm tactoe design). Shower the top with olive oil,

20. and afterward sprinkle with sesame and poppy seeds. Allow the mixture to ascend for 30 minutes more in a warm place.

21. Carefully lift the material paper with the batter, and put it on the st2 inside the stove. Prepare the bread for 40 minutes.

22. Remove the bread from the stove once cooked, and let it cool for around 30an hour prior to cutting it.

23. The bread is still a piece sticky in surface when hot and recently out of the oven.

Creamy Yogurt Fresh Fruit Salad

Ingredients:

- 2 cups grapes

- 1 8ounce compartment of vanilla or plain yogurt

- 1 teaspoon sugar

- 2 teaspoons lemon juice

- ½ teaspoon vanilla extract

- 2 cups strawberries, sliced

- 2 bananas, sliced

- 2 new peaches, sliced

- Lime juice

Directons:

1. Mix all the natural product together in a major bowl
2. Mix in around 3 tablespoons of lime juice to keep the natural products from going brown.
3. This likewise assists with supporting the flavor.
4. Mix yogurt, sugar, lemon juice, and vanilla in a little bowl.
5. You have the choice to either serve the yogurt blend as a plunge for the organic products, or blend it right in with the natural product to make a salad.
6. Serve right away

Quinoa Superfood Breakfast Bowl

Ingredients:

- 2 Medium whole banana sliced

- 1/2 Cup of blueberries fresh or frozen

- 1/2 Cup of Almond Milk (or a plantbased milk of your choice)

- 1/4 cup of walnuts

- ½ Cup plain cooked quinoa (or use mixed color if you prefer)

- 1 tbsp of peanut butter

Directons:

1. Combine quinoa and water in a small pot and bring to a boil.

2. Once boiling, cover pot with a lid and reduce heat to low.

3. Cook for around 15 minutes or until quinoa is cooked through. I cook extra and just store in the fridge.

4. Slice banana. Mix all Ingredients: together into a bowl and enjoy!

5. Serve warm or cold, so you can always cook the quinoa the night before if you'd prefer.

6. Serve warm or cold, which ever you prefer. I like both.

Almonds And Frozen Berry Oats

Ingredients:

- 3/4 cup of rolled oats

- 1/3 cup of unsweetened vanilla almond milk (use a brand of your choice)

- 1 tbsp of flax oil

- 1/4 cup of frozen berry mix

- 1/4 cup of almonds

- 1 tbsp of peanut butter or almond butter

- 1/4 cup of water

Directons:

1. Mix all Ingredients: into a big bowl (except for the frozen blueberries).

2. Cook in a microwave for about 34 minutes (cooking time vary from 2 microwave to another)
3. Stir the mix 2 minutes after cooking has started (so the mix doesn't stick or create chunks) .
4. Once the mix is cooked, add the frozen berry mix, and enjoy!

Banana Nut Bread

Ingredients:

- 1/4 teaspoon sea salt

- 1/2 cup raisins

- 1/2 cup chopped pecans

- 4 eggs

- 2 ripe bananas

- 1 1/2 cups unsweetened apple sauce

- 1/2 cup coconut milk

- 1 teaspoon vanilla

- 1/2 cup mixed nuts (for top)

- 1/2 cup almond flour

- 1 cup coconut flour

- 1/4 cup arrowroot powder

- 2 teaspoons cinnamon

- 2 teaspoons baking soda

Directions:

1. Line a 9" x 5" bread pan with parchment paper.
2. In a bowl, combine dry Ingredients:. Mix well.
3. Combine wet Ingredients: in a bowl. Mix well, using a a hand mixer.
4. Add dry Ingredients: to wet Ingredients:. Mix well using a a hand mixer.
5. Pour batter into the bread pan, and sprinkle the top with mixed nuts.
6. Bake in a preheated oven at 350 degrees for 6065 minutes. When toothpick comes out clean, remove from oven.

7. Toast, and serve topped with almond butter.

Breakfast Porridge

Ingredients:

- 3 tablespoons sunflower seeds

- 2 tablespoons ground flax seeds

- 1/2 teaspoon cinnamon

- Pinch of sea salt

- Optional toppings

- Dried fruit (raisins or chopped apricots)

- Cacao nibs

- 1 scoop nut butter

- 1 1/2 cups pureed pumpkin

- 2 1/2 tablespoons coconut flakes, fine shredded

- 2 tablespoons coconut cream

- 1 banana, mashed

- Crushed almonds (pecans, or walnuts)

Directions:

1. In a large bowl, combine all Ingredients:. Mix well.
2. Place in a small saucepan and warm over a low heat for 15 minutes, stirring frequently.
3. Add toppings as desired and serve.

Apple Hash Breakfast

Ingredients:

- 5 walnut, halves

- 1 1/2 tablespoons butter, grass fed

- 1 1/2 teaspoons cinnamon

- 2 eggs, beaten

- 3 slices bacon, cut into small strips

- 1 apple, peeled and chopped

Directions:

1. Scramble the eggs in the butter (in a large skillet). Remove.

2. Add bacon to the skillet and cook. When it's d2, add apple pieces and cook with the bacon until the apple is slightly soft.

3. Crush the walnuts and add to the apple and bacon.

4. Return the eggs to the skillet and stir all Ingredients: together.

5. Add the cinnamon to the mixture and stir.

Chicken Philly

Ingredients:

- ¼ cup white onions, sliced

- ½ teaspoon universally handy seasoning

- ½ teaspoon garlic powder

- 2 6inch entire wheat sub rolls

- 2 cuts without fat American cheese

- 1 b2less, skinless chicken bosom, cut into slight strips

- ¼ cup green ringer peppers, cultivated and cut

- 4 mushrooms

Directions:

1. Coat a skillet with nonstick shower and cook chicken fingers on mediumhigh hotness for 8 to 10 minutes.

2. Add peppers, onions, mushrooms, generally useful flavoring, and garlic powder to skillet.

3. Cook for extra 5 to 8 minutes on medium hotness or until chicken is completely cooked and veggies are browning.

4. Divide and scoop chicken and veggies into each roll.

5. Top hot blend with a cut of cheddar so it will dissolve inside the sandwich. Serve hot.

Slow Cooker French Coq Av Vin

Ingredients:

- 1½ teaspoons herbes de Provence

- 1½ teaspoons ocean salt

- 1½ teaspoons ground dark pepper

- 3 pounds b2less, skinless chicken thighs

- ½ pound solidified pearl onions, defrosted

- 8 ounces button mushrooms

- ½ cup tomato glue

- 2 tablespoons coconut flour

- 1 cup dry red wine or chicken soup

- 6 cuts bacon, coarsely hacked

- 2 huge cloves garlic, minced

Directions:

1. Coat a 5 to 6quart moderate cooker with cooking splash. In the pot, whisk the tomato glue with the coconut flour until the flour breaks down.
2. Whisk in the wine or soup, herbs, salt, and pepper until smooth.
3. Include the chicken, onions, mushrooms, bacon, and garlic.
4. Mix to coat the chicken with the sauce.
5. Cover and cook on high for 2½ to 3 hours or on low for 5 to 6.

Tasty Creamy Parmesan Chicken

Ingredients:

- 1 can (13.6 ounces) coconut milk

- 1 cup destroyed Gouda, Swiss, or Colby cheese

- ½ cup ground Parmesan cheese, isolated

- 4 b2less, skinless chicken breast parts

- 6 scallions, white and light green parts, meagrely cut

Directions:

1. Preheat the oven to 375°F. Coat a 9" × 9" heating dish with cooking shower.
2. Place the chicken in the dish.

3. Sprinkle with the scallions. In a medium dish, join the coconut milk, Gouda, Swiss, or Colby, and ¼ cup of the Parmesan.

4. Pour over the chicken mixture. Sprinkle with the remaining ¼ cup Parmesan.

5. Heat for 30 minutes, or until percolating and a thermometer embedded in the thickest segment registers 165°F and the juices run clear.

6. Let stand for 5 minutes prior to serving.

Sweet Peach Crisp

Ingredients:

- ½ tsp. vanilla concentrate

- 2 tbsp. Butter

- 1 ¼ c. almond flour, whitened

- Salt

- 1 kg. peaches, cut

- 1 tbsp. maple syrup

Directions:

1. Lay out the cut peaches into a heating dish. Blend the almond flour and salt in a sustenance processor.

2. At that point, beat with the butter, maple syrup, and vanilla.

3. Pour mixture over the peaches.

4. Prepare in the oven for roughly 45 minutes at 350 degrees.

5. Give it a chance to cool before serving.

Slow Cooker Chicken Cacciatore

Ingredients:

- 1 large red bell pepper, cored and sliced

- 1 (14.5ounce) can diced tomatoes

- 8 ounces sliced mushrooms

- ¾ teaspoon dried oregano

- ½ teaspoon dried basil

- 2 tablespoons olive oil

- 3 ½ to 4 lbs. whole chicken, cut into pieces

- 1/3 cup wholewheat flour

Directions:

1. Heat the oil in a large skillet over mediumhigh heat.

2. Toss the chicken with the flour and add it to the skillet – cook for 5 minutes on each side until browned.
3. Place the chicken in the bottom of the slow cooker and top with bell peppers, tomatoes, and mushrooms then sprinkle with herbs.
4. Cover the slow cooker and cook on low heat for 4 to 6 hours until the chicken is cooked through.

AlmondCrusted Baked Haddock

Ingredients:

- ½ cup wholewheat flour

- ¼ cup finely chopped almonds

- 1 tablespoon dried parsley

- 4 (6ounce) b2less haddock fillets

- Olive oil

- Fresh ground pepper

Directions:

1. Preheat the oven to 350°F and line a baking sheet with parchment.
2. Season the fillets with pepper and brush with olive oil.

3. Combine the whole wheat flour, almonds and parsley in a mixing bowl.
4. Sprinkle the mixture over the fish in a thick layer.
5. Bake for 10 to 12 minutes until the flesh flakes easily with a fork.
6. Serve the fillets hot with lemon wedges.

Onepot cabbage & beans with white fish

Ingredients:

- 2 celery sticks, diced

- 2 carrots , diced

- Small bunch thyme

- 1 savoy cabbage , shredded

- 4 tbsp white wine

- 300ml chicken stock

- Small knob of butter

- 5 rashers smoked streaky bacon , chopped

- 1 onion , finely chopped

- 410g can flageolet bean in water, drained

For the fish

- 2 tbsp plain flour

- 2 tbsp olive oil

- 4 fillets sustainable white fish , such as hake, about 140g/5oz each, skin on

Directions:

1. Heat the butter in a large sauté pan until starting to sizzle, add the bacon, then fry for a few mins.
2. Add the onion, celery and carrots, then gently cook for 810 mins until softening, but not brown.
3. Stir in the thyme and cabbage, then cook for a few mins until the cabbage starts to wilt.
4. Pour in the wine, simmer until evaporated, then add the stock and beans.

5. Season, cover the pan, then simmer gently for 10 mins until the cabbage is soft but still vibrant.

6. When the cabbage is d2, cook the fish.

7. Season each fillet, then dust the skin with flour.

8. Heat the oil in a frying pan. Fry the fish, skinside down, for 4 mins until crisp, then flip over and finish on the flesh side until cooked through.

9. Serve each fish fillet on top of a pile of cabbage with a few small potatoes, if you like.

Zesty haddock with crushed potatoes & peas

Ingredients:

- Juice and zest ½ lemon

- 1 tbsp capers, roughly chopped

- 2 tbsp snipped chives

- 4 haddock or other chunky white fish fillets, about 120g each (or use 2 small per person)

- 2 tbsp plain flour

- 600g floury potato, unpeeled, cut into chunks

- 140g frozen peas

- 2 ½ tbsp extravirgin olive oil

- Broccoli, to serve

Directions:

1. Cover the potatoes in cold water, bring to the boil, then turn to a simmer.
2. Cook for 10 mins until tender, adding peas for the final min of cooking.
3. Drain and roughly crush together, adding plenty of seasoning and 1 tbsp oil. Keep warm.
4. Meanwhile, for the dressing, mix 1 tbsp oil, the lemon juice and zest, capers and chives with some seasoning.
5. Dust the fish in the flour, tapping off any excess and season.
6. Heat remaining oil in a nonstick frying pan.
7. Fry the fish for 23 mins on each side until cooked, then add the dressing and warm through.
8. Serve with the crush and broccoli.